A HEALING COASTAL WALK

A meditative story to massage your body
and relax your mind

BOOKS IN THE NATUREBODY® SERIES

—

Walking in an Ancient Forest

Camping Under the Night Sky

Relaxing by a Waterfall

A Peaceful Winter Ski

Swimming in a Tropical Sea

A Healing Coastal Walk

Relaxing in the High Desert

A Spirited Mountain Hike

The complete
NatureBody® Connection
program is available at

www.aquaterramassage.com

A NATUREBODY® MASSAGE STORY

A Healing COASTAL WALK

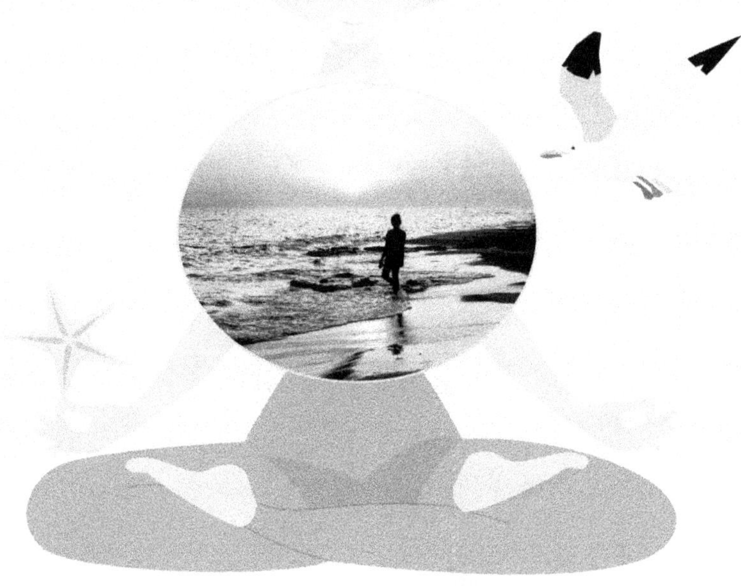

A meditative story to massage your body and relax your mind

ERIK KRIPPNER *and* FAYE KRIPPNER

Disclaimer: This book does not offer medical advice to the reader and is not intended as a replacement for appropriate healthcare and treatment. For such advice, readers should consult a licensed physician.

ISBN: 978-1-959772-01-9

Cover art provided by Envato Elements. Cover design by Faye Krippner and Erik Krippner.

Release Date for First Printed Edition 2023.

Media Inquiries: If you would like to contact the authors, please send an email to press@aquaterramassage.com.

Faye Krippner, B.A., LMT and Erik Krippner, B.S., LMT have been licensed by the Oregon Board of Massage Therapy since 2003. Oregon License Numbers: 10233 & 10234

Experience the entire NatureBody® Connection at
www.aquaterramassage.com

Dedicated to those who seek

to stretch their boundaries,

and to become one

with the sea and sky.

Index of Reflections

Contents

A WORD FROM THE AUTHORS

How to Use This Book

Humans have lived in balance with our bodies and the earth for 2.6 million years. Our bodies are designed for this planet. It is natural to walk on uneven ground, climb mountains, run long distances, swim, and most of all, to deeply breathe fresh air. Our wild planet heals and strengthens us by making us more flexible and fluid.

Your body is born of this earth. Earth is here to support you. Unfortunately, the stresses of life pull us off balance, and can leave us feeling physically sore and mentally anxious. This creative journey into relaxation is a way to remember your natural balance and create new muscle memories.

As massage therapists, we understand how a relaxed body feels: how it breathes, how it moves, how it is balanced in space. This NatureBody® massage story shares the full spectrum of massage: body, mind and spirit. Our intention is to empower you to find healing within yourself.

Visualization can have powerful effects on your body.[1] In this guided visualization, you will exercise your mind and imagination to deeply relax and bring your body back to center.

If you are injured or your ability to move is limited, then visualization is even more important! Studies have shown that when you imagine moving, the same areas of your brain activate as if you are actually moving those specific muscles.[2] Through visualization, you are virtually exercising your body.

We are intending for you to have a tangible, physical response to the ideas in this book. The power of this story lies in the vividness of your imagination. Read slowly. Pause. Use all of your senses to experience the story. Imagine the changes in humidity. Feel the gentle breeze on your skin. Hear the soothing sound of the wind. Smell the fresh scent of the life around you. Use your vibrant imagination to experience every detail in this story.

Put yourself in the story. Try to experience every sensation in your body. If you feel like moving, do it! Trust your instincts. Imagine what it feels like to move through the story: your muscles warming and stretching... your breathing deepening... your heartbeat slowing as you deeply relax. Let these sensations come to you at the speed of thought. This isn't about concentrating as much as it is about experiencing.

Each time you practice visualizing this story, your experience will become more vibrant. Your body is your wilderness to explore and understand. Your mind is your canvas for new muscle memories.

The Reflections are our personal notes to you. They offer you insight into some of the concepts in the story. Use them to spark your own creative thoughts about connection and healing.

The Notes section is full of wonderful articles and books that we have selected for you. If you feel interested in a topic, we highly recommend you look at the notes to explore the topic further.

The Journal at the end of the book gives you an opportunity to enhance and deepen your meditation. We have asked you a few thought-provoking questions to help you get started. Feel free to write or draw. Journal as creatively as you are inspired. This is your time to dream of the supportive connections between your body and nature.

There is much to discover about your relationship with your body and the beautiful world around you. Find a comfortable place to relax and enjoy. Prepare to be transported to a setting where you can unwind, immersed in nature, and experience the unbridled freedom of the wild!

From Wellness To Oneness,

Erik and Faye
Your Virtual Massage Therapists

FROM WELLNESS TO ONENESS

Wherever you are,
however you feel,
whatever your state of wellness,
know that
healing is at hand.

Your body is always seeking balance
and looking for opportunities to restore.

Through wellness,
may you come to oneness
with your body,
your mind,
your spirit,
and the beautiful Earth that supports us all.

ABOUT THIS MEDITATION

Introduction

Since early times, humans have been attracted to the seashore. Ancient peoples relied on the bounty of the ocean for decorative shells, vitamin-rich foods, and salt.

The ocean nourishes our body and nurtures our soul. We are soothed by the rhythmic sound of breaking waves. We witness the celestial power of the tides. Our mind calms as we breathe the sea air and gaze out to the horizon. The ocean rejuvenates our spirit and reignites our energy.

As waves crash and cool water runs up the beach, we are invigorated by a brisk walk at this border between sea and sky. Refresh your body and energize your spirit in this mindful walk by the ocean.

To experience the entire

NatureBody® Connection

scan this QR code

or go to

www.aquaterramassage.com / naturebodygift / coastalwalk

A gift for you, dear reader.

A special reading by the authors awaits you at the link above.

CHAPTER ONE

Over the Dunes

LEG MASSAGE FOR CIRCULATION

The wind blows steadily. Gray clouds parade across the sky. I am walking across the sand dunes on my way to the ocean. I take short strides as I climb the hills of soft sand. My feet slide backwards into little hollows they make with each step.

I walk slowly, giving my circulation time to establish itself through every capillary of my legs down to my toes. Walking in the soft, deep sand works my muscles completely. My legs rush with the heat of circulation. I feel energized.

My legs are expressing their primal purpose:
to move, to pump… to be strong and supple.

They feel long and limber
as they fulfill their purpose.

REFLECTION

Our Powerful Legs

"I am taking a ride on my powerful legs."

Our muscles are continually adapting to the challenges we give them. Our legs, in particular, enjoy moving. The more we use them, the stronger they get and the more fluid our motions feel. With strong legs, moving begins to feel like floating on a strong, supportive foundation.

Even if your mobility is limited, your body responds to your thoughts.[3] Imagine yourself walking powerfully. Visualize your legs moving strongly across the ground. Your strong thigh muscles engage as you propel yourself forward. Imagine the feeling of the breeze on your face and chest as you walk into the wind. Allow your breathing to free as you feel circulation coursing through you. As you visualize yourself walking, your brain is firing in the same patterns as if you were actually walking.[4] You are virtually giving yourself the experience of a satisfying walk.

The next time you go for a walk, notice your leg muscles working. Press each leg back a little farther, firing your glute muscles with every step. Feel the locomotion of your legs dependably moving in rhythm. You are becoming more fluid as you move: circulating breath, blood, and heat throughout your body.

Real or imagined, walking is a wonderful way to seek health. Your muscles flush with joy as they perform. They are becoming stronger for the walks to come, reveling in health.

I am taking a ride on my powerful legs.

They rhythmically carry me along to the beach.

I feel them becoming more vigorous and spirited
as they move strongly.

My long stride reaches from my abs.

I imagine my hips are extensions of my legs.
They swing in opposition to one another
to balance the ride of my stride.

My arms swing to balance the perpetual motion of this pace.

I feel the connection between my legs and spine
as my whole body participates in this walk.

My thighs and glutes are working hard,
helping my front hips to stretch and extend their reach.

My abdominal muscles engage
to keep me from leaning forward
and help me ride more buoyantly upon my hips.

REFLECTION

Circulation and Gravity

"As my leg muscles squeeze, they force deoxygenated blood back up, defying gravity with their strength."

Everything on our planet is subject to the laws of gravity: even our circulation. Unless encouraged upward, the fluid in our legs tends to pool down toward our ankles.

Our bodies rely on muscle contraction to help push fluid back up to our heart. The squeezing and releasing of muscles pumps circulation upwards against gravity. Valves in the veins of our legs prevent blood from falling back toward our feet.

In order to maximize the flow of circulation, your body requires two things of your leg muscles. First, your muscles need to squeeze strongly. Second, your muscles must release and relax between contractions.

To improve your circulation, stretch and massage your muscles. This helps them relax more fully, preparing for the next contraction. Exercise your legs to strengthen their ability to squeeze. Get up and dance! You can even sit and dance! Most of all, have fun! There are so many enjoyable and engaging activities for your legs.

As your legs pump, they are bringing circulation back up to your heart, keeping your body healthy and nourished.

I am walking tall and smooth.

Blood flows through my body
as the muscles of my legs pump strongly.

My powerful leg muscles
return circulation back up to my heart,
to be nourished and flow again.

As my leg muscles squeeze,
they force deoxygenated blood back up,
defying gravity with their strength.

I enter the meditation of walking.

Beach grasses have stabilized the shifting dunes, sheltering the landscape from high winds and storms.

Cresting the last hill, I am blasted by marine air. The vast ocean reveals itself from this vantage. I slide down the dunes and cross the beach to the ocean's edge.

CHAPTER TWO

Embrace of Sea and Sky

BREATHING AND GROUNDING

I stand tall, facing the ocean. Thick, silver-edged clouds mottle the daylight, bringing excitement to the day. The steady breeze fills my lungs with fresh sea air.

I put on my windbreaker, which shields me from the mist.

Looking down the coastline is absolutely stunning. Lush, green forested mountains pour down to the sand dunes that edge the beach. The slender, sandy beach is lined with huge driftwood logs that have made their way down from the forests and floated along the coastline before resting on the sand.

Traveling far from distant horizons, ocean winds build tiny ripples into statuesque ocean waves, which gallop to shore like the storied horses of Neptune. Winds amplify the energy of the majestic waves. The gray-blue sea churns into sharp white peaks.

REFLECTION

Energized Breathing

"This inspires me to exhale deeper, that I may fully enjoy my inhales."

Many of us do not pay attention to our breathing. Becoming aware of your breathing empowers you to be more energized as well as more relaxed with every breath. Breathing exercises free us from old habits and strengthen our respiratory muscles.

Normally, when we think about breathing, we focus on the inhale. This exercise reverses the active effort of breathing. Your exhales become active, and inhales, passive.

Try this breathing exercise. Imagine there is a powerful breeze that is blowing strongly into your nose and mouth. Instead of pulling the air into your body, relax and accept the inhale. Allow it to flow, using minimal effort.

On your exhale, push the air out against the pressure of the incoming breeze. Exhale completely, squeezing all the air out of your lungs. This exhale strengthens your diaphragm and abdominal muscles.

By changing the way you think about breathing, you can strengthen your respiratory muscles and become a stronger, more satisfied breather. A vigorous, healthy respiratory system gives you the energy and stamina to live more fully.

There is a constant blending of elements as waves break, and clouds bluster downwards. The sea and the sky reach toward one another in a wild embrace.

As chaotic seas churn, ozone is released into the salty air.

This fresh marine air races toward me.

I inhale deeply.

It rushes into my nostrils,
helping me take large, refreshing breaths.

I take another invigorating breath of cool marine air.

This inspires me to exhale deeper,
that I may fully enjoy my inhales.

I imagine the ocean air cleanses my body
of stagnant air and energy.

The steady breeze carries my exhales past my cheeks and ears and down the beach behind me.

My bare feet connect with the Earth.

I imagine drawing air in through my feet,
letting it whoosh up my body,
and spout out of the top of my head, like a whale.

My exhales absorb energy from above,
washing the power of the sky over my scalp,
neck,

REFLECTION

On Connection

"The idea of exchanging energy from above and below sensitizes me."

Your body constantly reacts and responds to the world around you. Temperatures, textures, sounds and scents intimately connect you to your environment. You are in a continual relationship with the ever-changing planet.

When we feel our connection to all that is around us, we become a part of something larger. The concept of something greater than ourselves is humbling. This sense of awe and reverence helps us become happier, more altruistic and less anxious.[5] To live with a sense of awe can be truly awesome.

Breathing can remind you of your sense of connection. Inhale. Imagine that you are pulling the air down from the sky. Draw it into the center of your body. Picture your breath pooling in your abdomen.

Exhale. Visualize your breath washing down your neck. Let it flow down your shoulders, down through your legs and into the earth.

Visualize your sense of awareness extending past your physical body: down through the earth and up to the sky. Feel your connection with all that is around you.

This energetic exercise grounds and centers your physical body. It helps you become more steadfast in the constantly changing world around you.

shoulders and arms,
down my legs,
returning to the sand.

The idea of exchanging energy from above and below
sensitizes me.

I sense my skin billowing with my inhales
and softening with my exhales.

My whole body breathes.

Clouds and ocean wave together in a complex dance, meeting in an atmospheric river of energy that is flowing onshore now. My breaths take in the dancing wind with each inhale, and create eddies as I exhale. The swirling wind uplifts my spirits and energizes my body.

I imagine myself energetically connected
to the center of the Earth.

I draw my breath up through the Earth,
feeling it fill me with its living, vital warmth.

Feeling connected, I beam it up to the sky.

I also receive energy from the sky,
drawing it down my body
and beaming it through the core of the Earth.
I feel grounded and centered.

CHAPTER THREE

Touch of the Ocean

FOOT AND CALF MASSAGE

Waves crash and fan up the sand. Each time the chilly saltwater slides over my toes, I feel a thrill up my spine. I skip and prance through the shallow beach waves. My feet relish the touch of the ocean on Earth.

Sea foam is set free from the receding water. It skitters and rolls with the wind past me. I exist within a turbulent gathering. It is exhilarating to walk between the clouds and the sea. I am drawn into the ever-changing story between the two.

The clouds and wind whip my hair as the ocean tickles my toes. Seawater laps at my ankles and the cuffs of my rolled up pants.

I am one with air and water.

REFLECTION

Walking Through Sand

"All of the muscles in my feet and calves respond to the changing viscosity of the sand. Each step feels unique."

Your feet: two small miracles at the foundation of your body. The versatile muscles of your feet activate to support you in your activities. Whether you are walking, skipping, jumping, or dancing, your feet keep you balanced and upright.

Beach walking is a wonderful way to strengthen your feet.[6] Your pliable feet respond to the ground underneath them. They move differently when you are walking on a hard surface versus soft soil. When you walk in soft sand, every step is unique. Your feet respond to the shifting sand, muscularly pressing forward as sand slides underneath them.

There are many muscles in your feet: muscles that arch and curl your feet, and spread and wiggle your toes. You can practice strengthening these muscles by picking up a pencil or a sock with your toes.

Here is another exercise for your feet. Place a hand towel on the floor and rest the ball of your foot on the near edge of the towel. Keeping your heel on the ground, pull the towel evenly back toward you by curling your toes and arch. Once you have gathered the towel underneath your foot, push the towel forward, inch by inch, until it is flat in front of you again.

Challenging your feet with new activities helps them become stronger and more versatile.[6]

I walk easily and fluidly across smooth, wetly packed sand.

My feet tingle as they are stimulated
by the cool seawater,
the texture of the sand,
and the breeze blowing on my wet skin.

I head upwind along the beach. In the distance ahead of me, a mountain ridge reaches into the ocean.

My feet leave imprints as they sink into the soft sand.

All of the muscles in my feet and calves respond
to the changing viscosity of the sand.

Each step feels unique.

My feet begin to feel more dynamic and open,
as if they have more talent and ability than I realize.

My foot widens as I press into the soft sand.

My toes reach
while my arch curls and cups the sand.

My feet are working like dolphin tails.

They feel like intelligent fins,
propelling me across the sand
as if they were swimming over it.

REFLECTION

On Hamstrings

"My hamstrings and glutes are able to express their strength as they pump strongly, propelling me forward in the soft sand."

Walking is a coordinated dance of muscular effort. All of the muscles in our legs work together to move us forward, while keeping us balanced on our feet. When these muscles work in concert, they support our knees. If one of these muscle groups gets too tight or weak, however, our knees can get sore[7] and our stride less efficient.

Many of us who have experienced knee pain share a common imbalance. The muscles in the front of our thighs (our quadriceps muscles) are strong and overpower the back of our legs (our hamstring muscles).[8] This imbalance of strength causes our pelvis to tilt forward. To rebalance, we must stretch our quads and strengthen our hamstrings.

To strengthen the backs of your legs and hips, lengthen your stride. Squeeze your glutes to pull your leg back when you walk.[9] Your hamstrings and glutes fire to launch you forward powerfully while keeping your upper body upright. As your hamstrings and glute muscles become stronger, they help tilt your pelvis upright, allowing you to walk taller.

Squats are another effective way to strengthen your hamstrings.[10] If you are just getting started, use a table or chair to help balance while you become comfortable deeply bending your knees with an upright back.

When the muscles of your legs and hips are balanced, they work in harmony to move you efficiently and protect your joints.

The calf muscles of my lower legs conduct
the harmonious rhythms and dance of my feet.

They warm as they squeeze,
and the effort soon travels up my legs.

I bend my knees deeply as I walk,
and my hamstrings and glutes are able
to express their strength as they pump strongly,
propelling me forward in the soft sand.

My stride becomes more fluid.

I picture myself floating above the sand,
like a jellyfish:
an angelic moon,
pulsing and pumping effortlessly in the ocean.

I imagine my walk,
floating and pulsing
as if I were weightless.

The lower I breathe in my body,
the more buoyant I feel.

My legs fall into a comfortable cadence.

I am moving with the breath and beat of the ocean,
accented by the crashing surf.

CHAPTER FOUR

The Vista

FULL BODY MEDITATION

My long walk brings me closer to the end of this beach. Ahead of me, a forested mountain ridge reaches out into the sea. As I get closer, the wind subsides in the protection of the ridge.

A trail zigzags up the hill. The narrow path passes through abundant, hardy coastal shrubs with waxy leaves and woody stems, called salal. Salal fortifies the mountainside, and stabilizes the trail.

Winding my way up the steep, sandy path,
circulation courses through my body.

I find my feet sliding a bit.

REFLECTION

Walking Uphill

"My arms and legs both work in time
to propel me up the slope."

Simple, coordinated, and sustained exercises like walking can revitalize your body, mind and spirit.

Walking is a wonderful, full-body activity. Because it is a low-impact exercise, walking builds your bones without putting a lot of impact on your joints. It strengthens your legs, hips, and core muscles to support and stabilize your spine.[11]

Walking uphill is particularly wonderful, because it exercises the muscles in the back of your legs[12] and helps balance your pelvis. A balanced pelvis frees the stride of your legs and is the foundation for a healthy spine.

To maximize the positive effects of walking, it is important to keep good form. Stand up tall. Look ahead of you, not at the ground. Visualize floating your core across the earth. Maintaining good posture supports your spine.

When we walk, our legs and arms swing in opposite cadence. These alternating, full-body movements promote circulation through our whole body. They also fortify our sense of balance and coordination. Walking brings our brain into a "happy state" by releasing the feel-good chemicals, dopamine, norepinephrine and serotonin.[13]

Walking is a simple exercise that carries tremendous benefits for our whole being.

Some sections of the trail
are softer and steeper than others.

My arms and legs both work in time
to propel me up the slope.

The trail becomes firmer as the sand becomes soil.

My stride feels quick and powerful
as I walk through this solid terrain.

The trail winds through a grove of shore pines, each uniquely contorted and shaped by strong sea winds. Their strength and zeal for life have allowed them to find fresh water on these salty shores and grow strong enough to hold the mountainside together, slowing erosion.

The path levels as I reach the spine of the ridge. I feel the excitement of this new milestone and relief from the wind as I walk through the protection of the trees. The spice of evergreen welcomes my return to the lush, coastal forest.

At the end of the ridge, a rocky prominence offers an uninterrupted vista. I am far above the water, and the crashing of the surf is muted. The wind has eased. I feel calm and relaxed here.

The ocean looks more serene from this height. I enjoy the patterns of the waves reverberating off the headlands. They crisscross, fanning away through the incoming ocean rollers.

The huge gray-blue clouds that have been rolling through the sky all day have broken apart and settled into a field of puffy cotton ball clouds.

REFLECTION

On Whale Spouts and Breathing

"A whale spouts in the distance."

When a whale surfaces, it has only a couple of seconds to exchange the air in its massive lungs. It forcefully exhales with an energetic spout. Then it inhales fully before diving back into the ocean.

The whale's powerful exhale empties most of the stagnant air from its body, making its inhale more replenishing. Whales exchange 80-90% of the air in their bodies with each breath.[14]

In contrast, humans exchange about 10-15% of the air in our lungs. We can increase our lung capacity by taking a lesson from the whale. If we exhale fully, we can increase the amount of oxygen we intake with each breath.[15] A strong exhale invites a more complete inhale.

As you walk, breathe like a whale. Exhale energetically, forcing all the air out of your lungs. Allow your next, cleansing inhale to replenish your lungs with a full, deep breath.

While we will never be as efficient as a whale, there are humans who have held their breath for 24 minutes.[16] Your goal may not be to hold your breath, but you can develop the strength and technique to achieve a more satisfying breath. Breathe deeply, so you can think clearly, relax fully, and have the energy to do the things you love.

From up here, the sky is balanced in proportion to the sea.

I, too, feel balanced.

My lungs have breathed this sky
and my feet have danced at the edge of this ocean.

I breathe slowly,
my warm muscles singing
in a whole body glow.

A whale spouts in the distance. As the sun drops through the clouds, a pink glow illuminates this tranquil world.

I watch the calming seas,
and I feel my own body continuing to calm.

My pulse has slowed.
My body feels delightfully warm.

My shoulders are relaxed and heavy
and slide down my long, supported spine.

My jaw is relaxed.

My mind is quiet as I watch
the tranquility of the sea.

CHAPTER FIVE

Gratitude

A BLESSING FROM THE OCEAN

Thank you for joining me on this hike today. Since humans have walked this planet, we have been drawn to the ocean, our ancient home.

May the power of water
cleanse your soul and buoy your spirit.

May the strength of wind
dance in your soul and inspire you to new heights.

May the fiery warmth of your legs
keep you circulating over this beautiful planet.

May the Earth, which holds oceans,
reveal the strength which lies in you.

Dream on, Tranquil Wanderer. Until we meet again.

Acknowledgments

My grandmother, Betty Erickson, brought me on memorable walks along the Oregon coastline throughout my childhood. Her playful spirit travels with me to this day.

We are grateful to Clark and Kyra Rogerson, and for the wonderful times we have had at the coast together, watching ships sail over the ocean and storms roll across the sky.

We enjoyed learning about marine weather patterns from Lee Chesneau, author of *Heavy Weather Avoidance and Route Design: Concepts and Applications of 500Mb Charts*. Lee explained how weather systems move over the oceans, and taught us how to read the surface and 500MB ocean analyses. His brief lessons have helped us to read the weather for ourselves.

Thank you to Tim Thomsen of San Juan Kayak Expeditions for a beautiful experience of connecting with the sea from the vantage of a kayak. We were blessed to witness orcas and their baby calves swimming right under our boat.

Notes

1. "What is Imagery?" *Johns Hopkins Medicine*, 2003, www.hopkinsmedicine.org/health/wellness-and-prevention/imagery.

2. Lohr, Jim. "Can Visualizing Your Body Doing Something Help You Learn to Do It Better?" *Scientific American*, 1 May 2015, www.scientificamerican.com/article/can-visualizing-your-body-doing-something-help-you-learn-to-do-it-better.

3. Hampton, Debbie. "How Your Thoughts Change Your Brain, Cells and Genes." *Huffington Post*, 23 March 2016, www.huffpost.com/entry/how-your-thoughts-change-your-brain-cells-and-genes_b_9516176.

4. Niles, Frank. "How to Use Visualization to Achieve Your Goals." *Huffington Post*, 17 June 2011, www.huffpost.com/entry/visualization-goals_b_878424.

5. Allen, Summer. "Eight Reasons Why Awe Makes Your Life Better." *Greater Good Magazine*, 26 September 2018, greatergood.berkeley.edu/article/item/eight_reasons_why_awe_makes_your_life_better.

6. Cadman, Bethany. "What Are the Best Foot Exercises for Healthy Feet?" *Medical News Today*, 16 April 2021, www.medicalnewstoday.com/articles/320964.

7. "Knee Pain." *Mayo Clinic*, www.mayoclinic.org/diseases-conditions/knee-pain/symptoms-causes/syc-20350849. Accessed 3 February 2023.

8. Hughes, Cody. "What Is 'Quad Dominance' and Why Does it Affect Almost Everyone?" *Stack Sports*, 23 July 2019, www.stack.com/a/quad-dominance-what-it-is-and-why-it-affects-almost-everyone.

9. Beverly, Jonathan. "It's All in the Hips." *Runners World*, 31 March 2014, www.runnersworld.com/advanced/a20847674/its-all-in-the-hips.

10. Chertoff, Jane. "What Muscles Do Squats Work?" *Healthline*, 23 May 2019, www.healthline.com/health/exercise-fitness/what-muscles-do-squats-work.

11. "Walking for Exercise and Spine Health." *Nebraska Spine Health*, 22 April 2021, nebraskaspinehospital.com/walking-exercise-spine-health.

12. Lovett, Richard. "Hike to Stronger Hamstrings." *Outside Magazine*, 6 March 2020, www.outsideonline.com/health/running/training-advice/workouts/hike-to-stronger-hamstrings.

13. Laurence, Emily. "The Best Underrated Exercise for Keeping Your Brain Sharp Well Into Your 80s." *Well and Good*, 29 June 2022, www.wellandgood.com/exercise-and-brain-health.

14. Berry, George. "How Do Whales Breathe?" *Whale and Dolphin Conservation,* 20 October 2012, us.whales.org/2012/10/20/how-do-whales-breathe.

15. Polatin, Betsy. "Breath in Motion: Why Exhaling Matters Most." *Huffington Post,* 21 February 2014, www.huffpost.com/entry/breath-in-motionwhy-exhal_b_4769819.

16. Suggitt, Connie. "56-Year-Old Freediver Holds Breath for Almost 25 Minutes Breaking Record." *Guinness World Records,* 12 May 2021, www.guinnessworldrecords.com/news/2021/5/freediver-holds-breath-for-almost-25-minutes-breaking-record-660285.

MEDITATION

Journal

This journal gives you a place to reflect on your experience as you read and meditate. With every meditation, your library of personal affirmations can grow. Some thoughts you might want to record, in words or drawings, are:

What were your favorite phrases or ideas in the story? How did you feel as you imagined walking along the coastline? What emotions did the blustery day invoke in you?

What breathing exercises have you learned over the years? Which ones do you still practice?

Describe your time by the water. What textures did you walk on? Soft or coarse sand? Rock? Clay? Grass? How did your feet, legs, and low back feel as you walked along the shore?

Talk about the times when you have felt the most energized. Which outdoor settings energize you? Which activities give you energy?

"I AM MOVING WITH THE BREATH AND BEAT OF THE OCEAN, ACCENTED BY THE CRASHING SURF."

MEDITATION

There is rhythm in the world around us and within us. From the tidal pull of the oceans, to the circulation coursing through our veins, we are part of the rhythmic song of the Earth.

~

"THE WIND RUSHES UNDER MY ARMS AND LIFTS ME UP."

MEDITATION

When the wind blows, it can influence the way you move and the way you feel. Wind in your face can bring tears to your eyes, delivering you completely to the present moment.

When wind blows on your chest, you lean into it, moving more powerfully to make progress. When you lift your arms, it rushes under them, creating an uplifting feeling as though you had wings.

Wind transforms the stillness of nature into a tangible flow of energy.

~

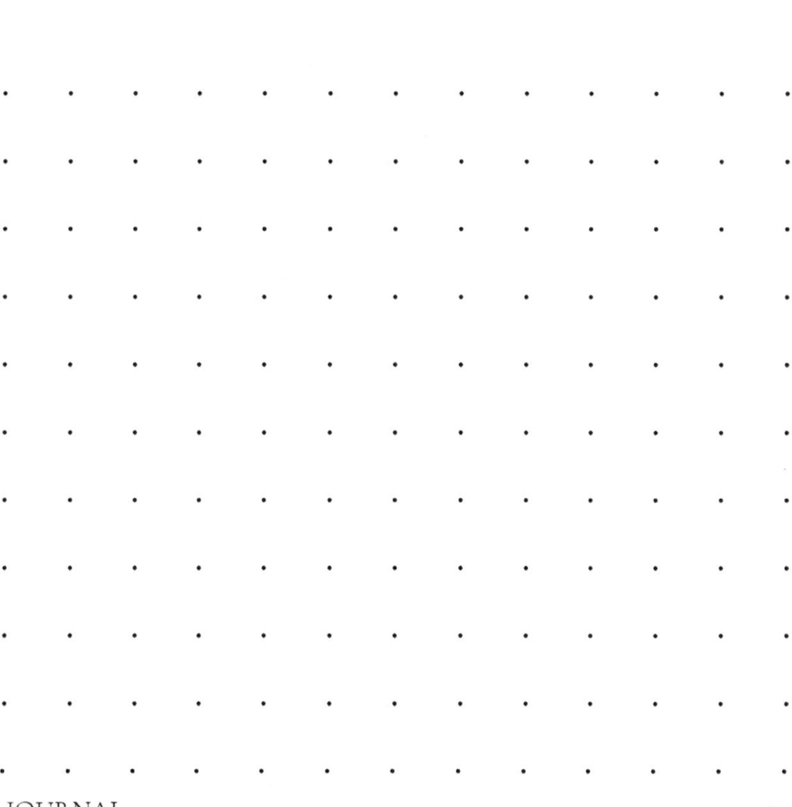

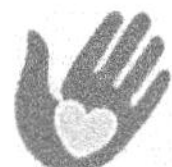

May the

POWER

of

WATER

cleanse your soul

and buoy your spirit.

"AS THE SUN DROPS THROUGH THE CLOUDS, A PINK GLOW ILLUMINATES THE WATERY WORLD."

Close your eyes and imagine a glorious sunset. Appreciate the refraction of light through Earth's atmosphere. With each second that passes, sunset transforms, its colors and textures ever-changing, until the last rays disappear under the horizon. These moments of singular beauty remind us how precious it is to be here, now.

~

"MY LUNGS HAVE BREATHED THIS SKY AND MY FEET HAVE DANCED AT THE EDGE OF THIS OCEAN."

MEDITATION

As you walk your life's path across the planet, you create experiences with Earth. With every breath and every step, your relationship with the planet deepens.

How have you deepened your relationship with the planet today?

~

May the

STRENGTH

of

WIND

dance in your soul

and inspire you

to new heights.

"IT IS EXHILARATING TO WALK BETWEEN THE CLOUDS AND THE SEA. I AM DRAWN INTO THE EVER-CHANGING STORY BETWEEN THE TWO."

MEDITATION

We live on the boundary between great forces: we walk the border between earth and air, and we swim at the meniscus of water and sky. There is a unique blending of elements at the ocean. Wind waves the ocean, churning the water upward into the sky. The air becomes infused with seawater, and the ocean bubbles and froths with air. It is a privilege to be a part of the relationship where great elements meet.

~

"THE MUSCLES IN MY FEET AND CALVES RESPOND TO THE CHANGING VISCOSITY OF THE SAND."

In the natural world, our bare feet conform to the earth when we walk. They reach and grip the ground. As the sand slides under our feet, our muscles get a thorough workout.

With strong, pliable feet, we move fluidly over the Earth.

~

May the

FIERY

WARMTH

of your legs

keep you circulating

over this beautiful planet.

"TRAVELING FAR FROM DISTANT HORIZONS, OCEAN WINDS BUILD TINY RIPPLES INTO STATUESQUE OCEAN WAVES, WHICH GALLOP TO SHORE LIKE THE STORIED HORSES OF NEPTUNE."

MEDITATION

The great and powerful waves of the ocean began as tiny ripples. What ripples of possibility exist in your life right now? How can you nurture your aspirations to encourage them to build and flourish?

~

"MY WHOLE BODY BREATHES, AS IF I CAN FEEL MY SKIN BILLOWING AND SOFTENING WITH MY BREATH."

MEDITATION

Close your eyes and feel the sensations of breathing. What do you notice?

~

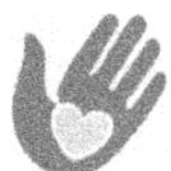

May the

EARTH,

which holds oceans,

reveal the strength

which lies in you.

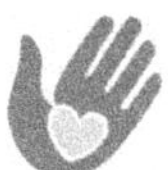

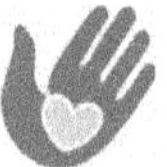

"MY JAW IS RELAXED AND MY THOUGHTS ARE PEACEFUL AS I WATCH THE TRANQUILITY OF THE SEA."

MEDITATION

Our bodies mirror what we see in the world around us. Find the tranquility in your surroundings and allow it to influence your body. Relax the focus of your vision to see a broader picture and allow your mind to enter a new level of awareness.

~

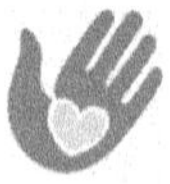

"MY FEET BEGIN TO FEEL MORE DYNAMIC AND OPEN, AS IF THEY HAVE MORE TALENT AND ABILITY THAN I REALIZE."

It can take a lot of training to become good at something, but along the way, it is the miracle of our bodies that actually connects the dots. There is a great deal of movement and coordination involved in the most basic of activities. Watch your body move as you perform a simple action. It seems to know what to do, without conscious thought. Be grateful for not having to think out every movement. Reflect on your miraculous body.

~

BLESSING
FROM THE OCEAN

May the

POWER OF WATER

cleanse your soul and buoy your spirit.

May the

STRENGTH OF WIND

dance in your soul and inspire you to new heights.

May the

FIERY WARMTH

of your legs
keep you circulating over this beautiful planet.

May the

EARTH,

which holds oceans,
reveal the strength which lies in you.

About the Authors

Born and raised in New Orleans, Erik Krippner grew up with a po'boy in his hand and a song in his heart. As a boy, he spent his summers swimming, hiking, fishing, and sailing. After becoming an Eagle Scout, Erik dreamed of answering the call to "Go West, young man." He earned a Bachelor of Science degree in Forestry from Louisiana State University. Following his passion for adventure, Erik found his way to the mountains of the Pacific Northwest, his home to this day. After working in the forests of Oregon, Washington, Idaho, Alaska, Georgia, and Louisiana, Erik decided to focus his love of natural sciences on the study of human body through massage therapy.

Faye grew up in Oregon surrounded by family and old growth coastal forests. She spent many childhood weekends cross-country skiing, hunting for mushrooms, exploring coastal tide pools, and searching for crawdads in the Siuslaw River. Her love of books deepened when she became the editor of her high school and college's literary journals. Upon earning her Bachelor of Arts degree in Mathematics with honors from the Robert D. Clark Honors College at the University of Oregon, Faye became a technical writer and web developer. The whisper of a deeper purpose ignited her to study massage, where she met Erik.

Erik and Faye became friends in massage school at the East West College of the Healing Arts, in Portland, Oregon. In 2003, they founded Aqua Terra Massage, a therapeutic massage studio for friends and couples. Since then, they have practiced therapeutic massage together, side by side. They have spent years immersed in the study of massage, serving thousands of clients.

Faye and Erik have spent years exploring and writing about our beautiful world. They have sailed the blue waters of Fiji's Koro Sea, kayaked New Zealand's Marlborough Sound, and stargazed among the giraffes and elephants in Botswana. They have hiked the Appalachian Trail and paddled the tidally-influenced Columbia River in the Pacific Northwest. They have seen orca whales swim right under their kayaks, locked eyes with wild lions, and played hide-and-seek with an octopus. They have hiked thousands of miles together, kayaked and sailed hundreds, and spent countless evenings camping under the stars.

With a commitment to bringing more love and kindness to this beautiful world, we offer this book to you.

www.aquaterramassage.com

www.ingramcontent.com/pod-product-compliance
Lightning Source LLC
Chambersburg PA
CBHW071035050426
42335CB00050B/1686

9781959772019